Neuroathletics training for beginners

More coordination, agility and concentration thanks to improved neuroathletics - incl. 10-week plan for training in everyday life.

Sebastian Borchert

CONTENT

What you can expect in this book

Do you feel that your training progress is stagnating? Are you looking for new stimuli that will benefit both your body and your mind? Do you want to get back into your sport after an injury or are you just starting to look for the activity that suits you and want to build an optimal routine?

Whether you are a professional athlete or an amateur, neuroathletic training is suitable for everyone and capable of immensely supporting the progress of each individual. This created since the advance of some sports scientists a few years ago, a completely new perspective on the causes of athletic success and the maximum exploitation of their own potential. The great advantage: there is no risk of injury, nor do you have to worry about making mistakes.

However, it's not just about pure performance enhancement in sports, but also about aspects that we need every day in everyday life: Coordination, agility, concentration. You will also learn to perform movements more consciously and thus prevent or alleviate pain.

Dive into the world of neuroscience, learn how our brain works and why we are able to move the way we do in the first place. Numerous exercises exist that will challenge you, but are just as fun, and will help you take your workout to a new level. The 10-week plan included in the book will guide you along the way and show you how you, too, can benefit from neuroathletic training - without a trainer. What are you waiting for? Start promoting your brain in a more targeted way - your body will thank you for it.

What is meant by neuroathletics training?

The classic view of athletic progress is probably familiar to everyone: We expose our bodies to certain stimuli and sequences of movements, repeat them regularly, and then continuously increase ourselves in order to be able to maintain the level and improve bit by bit. If we then look at ourselves in the mirror, see the progress and notice our new strength, we usually have our strained muscles, joints and tendons in the back of our minds when we think about how we were able to achieve this in the first place.

But we often forget one important factor: our nervous system with our brain as the control center. This controls every single movement we perform. Unfortunately, this also means that a large part of our training depends on it: The brain basically evaluates every situation according to whether it could be dangerous for us or not.

So if our nervous system delivers inaccurate or even too little information to the brain, it automatically initiates more cautious movements because it assumes a possible threat. It reduces the output of performance in order to prevent injuries. However, since we are not aware of this evaluation process and therefore cannot control it, we may unconsciously stand in our own way - regardless of whether we are descending a steep slope on a snowboard or performing a few stretching exercises on our yoga mat at home. You can think of it as similar to technical devices: The hardware (in this case our body) may be as stable and robust as it is - if the software has weak points and hangs or doesn't execute commands properly, it bothers us immensely.

And it is precisely this weak point that neuroathletic training addresses. This is based primarily on findings from neuroscience and enables a targeted influence on our nervous system by addressing and promoting our three movement-controlling instances. As a result, they are able to gather and transmit higher quality information so that the brain can safely recognize when we are safe and thus use our full power. It will now no longer intervene in a precautionary way, but will additionally help you to perform the desired movements in a safer and more focused way.

Especially in the aftermath of a previous injury, neuroathletics training is of great importance, as it can help you release unconscious blocks and regain your old strength. Your brain wants to do everything in its power to prevent you from sustaining further injuries in the future as a result of this painful event, so it will take much higher safety precautions when you start playing sports again. Overcoming these is almost impossible without training our nervous system. The idea is to bypass this automatic protective mechanism by using neuro-exercises to briefly switch off the particular area in the brain that was sending this unpleasant stimulus during the movement previously associated with pain. The exercise is then repeated painlessly and, above all, slowly to accustom the brain to the fact that this movement no longer poses a danger to the body. Before this process is complete, however, usually 80 hours of training must be completed. Neuroathletics should therefore be performed on a long-term basis and on a regular basis.

Neuroathletic training (also known as Neuro Athletic Training, or NAT for short) has been significantly shaped by sports scientist and trainer Lars Lienhard, who has been pursuing this training approach since 2010 and has made it known throughout Europe. In doing so, he incorporates the approaches of leading neuroathletics expert Dr. Eric Cobb, who already focuses on neuro-centered training and therapies with his "Z-Health" program. The Z stands for the Russian word "zdorovje," which means health. Cobb incorporated many different approaches and techniques into this training concept, but probably the most significant idea behind it is the consideration of the physiological impact of fear on our bodies. This brings us back to the question that influences everything: *"Could this situation be dangerous for me, if not threaten my life, or am I safe?"*

Lienhard has already used NAT to train various top athletes extremely effectively, for example coaching the German national team at the World Cup in Brazil in 2014 or the German track and field athletes at the Summer Olympics in 2016. The successful sprinter Gina Lückenkemper also benefits from NAT units.

This illustrates the effectiveness of this still new training approach. Contrary to the initial difficulties in getting it accepted and recognized in the entrenched view of the sports world, Lienhard was so successful with it that he was able to bring even the most trained athletes to a completely new level. Who would have even guessed beforehand what effects these small, sometimes strange-seeming exercises really have?

Let's look at an example: A middle-aged man exercises regularly with his body weight and knows what form to maintain during certain exercises in order to perform the movement cleanly. Nevertheless, he notices how he keeps slipping into bad postures because he lacks stability. He now wonders what he can do to train healthier and more effectively. If he were to seek the advice of several trainers or physical therapists, many would certainly advise him to incorporate stability training into his routine and to better develop his deep muscles. For example, forearm supports, lunges, or standing balances would be on the daily schedule to strengthen the core of the body in particular. But these exercises once again focus on the muscles. If we now look at the problem of instability in the context of neuroathletics training, completely new approaches to solutions arise in practice: trainers would have our amateur athlete snort here, for example.

What sounds very bizarre at first has a very simple

background: If you hold your nostril closed, then sniff and try to draw in as much air as possible, you activate a certain area of the brain. This area controls our head, eyes and spine and enables us to perform movements more stably and safely when it is actively engaged.

And that was just one example of many. For almost every problem that occurs during individual training - regardless of the type of sport or exercise practiced - you can find at least one exercise in NAT that can help you overcome it. Even if you have tried everything humanly possible and have not seen any significant improvement. In the end, it all comes down to one principle: if faulty or expandable processes are playing out in the brain, you can't make much progress physically, no matter how hard you work towards it. Fortunately, this applies equally to every single person, which is why everyone can benefit from neuroathletics training. So don't be put off by it if you haven't heard much about it before and now read that it's being used more and more in professional sports - there's always room for improvement, after all, even among athletes.

They have a completely different approach to training, they are guided by experts and the exercises are perfectly adapted to the requirements of their respective sport and their own unique neuroprofile.

However, since the tasks are very varied and, above all, easy to apply, there is also something for your progress. And the good thing is that there is no risk for you. Unlike, for example, deadlifts, where you can get extremely painful injuries to your back if you do them incorrectly, you can't do anything wrong with NAT, where also? Sniffing or exercises where you balance on a towel or cover your eye never hurt anyone. So don't be afraid to try it out, it can only work to your advantage!

The bridge between science and sport

But, before we talk about practice, let's first look at what athletes can learn from neuroscience.

This covers a broad range of topics that extends across the entire natural sciences: Due to the diverse methods neuro scientific research is conducted in biology, psychology, mathematics or even computer science, among others. The common denominator of all of them is research into the structure and functioning of nervous systems of all kinds. Their role in all life processes of biological organisms and how these can be reproduced and also imitated (among other things by technology) is therefore being investigated.

The tasks of our human nervous system can be roughly divided into three aspects:

1. Bundle the information from all our sensory organs, so this includes all internal and external influences.

2. These must then be considered in aggregate, primarily in terms of whether or not the situation at hand could threaten our survival and security.

3. Depending on the answer, an action decision must now be made. This usually results in the execution of movements.

Example: Your body registers that your so-called hunger center in the hypothalamus is releasing hormones and blood sugar is dropping. It now evaluates this development as hunger and signals the body that it is time to eat again. If the situation is now safe and there is no apparent threat in your environment, it makes the decision to eat. Consequently, you go to a food source, such as your home kitchen, and specifically make the movements you need there: Arrange already precooked food on a plate, heat it up in the microwave, take the plate, bring the fully loaded fork to your mouth and finally eat.

The research fields of neuroscience, which deal specifically with the functioning of the brains of primates, i.e. monkeys and humans, are summarized in general language under the term brain research. Neuroathletic training is also based on this.

The fascination with the functioning of the human brain goes back more than 5000 years. A number of findings in Egypt document the performance of surgical interventions in the central nervous system, which were hoped to provide answers to the many unanswered questions at the time. In addition to basic research per se, brain research is also conducted from other perspectives: for knowledge about causes and possible cures for nervous diseases such as Parkinson's and dementia, for understanding the neuronal processes involved in our perception, or even for the development of emotions. Philosophical phenomena such as the concept of consciousness are also addressed.

Our brain is a small marvel, consisting of about 100 billion nerve cells, the so-called neurons. These are in constant exchange with each other and send information via more than 100 trillion synapses to the responsible areas of the brain. Like a command center, it controls every single aspect of our existence: the subconscious processes such as breathing or blinking, the expression of our individual character traits, or even the management of external circumstances from our environment. We can orient ourselves, communicate with other people in different languages and we know how to adapt to diverse circumstances.

Although brain research has been going on for centuries, significant progress has been made in recent years. This has largely been achieved by two factors: on the one hand, the ever-growing knowledge of molecular biological processes and, on the other hand, the further development of imaging techniques such as CT or MRI. These enable scientists to measure the processes in the brain on the basis of increased blood flow to certain areas and greater metabolic activity, and then to display them three-dimensionally on a computer. Since the brain can basically be watched live while it thinks, conclusions can be drawn about how, for example, movement control or even the use of our language works. What an enormous development this represents becomes even clearer when one considers that brain research 150 years ago still had to make do with the information obtained from the autopsy of deceased persons and the analysis of dead brains.

The concrete effects that sport has on our brain have already been the subject of numerous studies. It helps us relieve stress and take a breather from the problems and worries of everyday life. Our brains are primarily focused on executing our movements correctly, and because we want to get the most out of our workouts, we don't allow unwanted thoughts to creep in. Simpler things come into focus: what equipment we're using, what exercise to do next, what route to take on today's run, or even the next move during volleyball practice. This gives us the opportunity to approach mental challenges with renewed vigor after the end of our training. When the focus shifts from physical exercise back to our everyday problems, we can look at them in a more detached way. If you were previously stuck in your mindset with no solution in sight, you may now come up with something you wouldn't have thought of before. Simply because you could hardly think clearly due to all the stress - you know the saying: Sometimes you can't see the forest for the trees.

A group of neuroscientists from Ulm, led by Susanna Stroth, investigated the further consequences of exercise. They had young adults complete an endurance running training program that lasted several weeks. The result: visual-spatial memory and the ability to concentrate were improved. Regular running also had a positive effect on the subjects' mood.

But these are not the only benefits of regular exercise: many different hormones are released, which help us control weight, prevent diseases or even build muscle. An interesting example of a hormone that particularly targets our brain would be the still very little known peptide YY. Even though the exact relationship between physical activity and its release is not yet completely known, studies have already proven that endurance training significantly raises our peptide YY levels. This has a particular effect on the brain areas responsible for controlling our hunger and appetite. As a result, we become full faster and feel less hungry after our workout.

Furthermore, the brain is better supplied with oxygen through exercise, which stimulates the formation of new brain cells. Concentration, performance and our memory are improved and fatigue is prevented. If we now exercise regularly, the brain gets used to the better blood flow over time, which in turn promotes the connections between the cells. In addition, growth hormones are released, which acts like a rejuvenating cure. Serotonin and dopamine give us feelings of happiness and reward, motivating us to keep going.

We can therefore conclude that there is a positive interaction between the brain and physical activity: our brain enables us to make the movements and helps us to perform them optimally, and the activity in turn keeps our brain fit and increases its performance. If we start there with neuroathletics training, we can further strengthen this effect, because the brain is trained specifically and not merely as a result of our daily life.

The three movement controlling instances

Neuroathletic training focuses in particular on the three movement-controlling instances of our nervous system: self-awareness, the sense of balance and the eyes together with the visual pathway.

So let's take a look at the basics of our motor actions.

THE PROPRIOCEPTIVE SYSTEM

Among experts, self-awareness is referred to as the proprioceptive system (from Latin: proprius = own, recipere = to receive). In contrast to the other two instances, it cannot be clearly localized because it does not belong to a specific sensory organ. Rather, self-awareness takes place via numerous receptors (proprioceptors) that are distributed throughout the body. They are found, for example, in joint capsules, tendons, muscles and ligaments. Another point of differentiation is that impressions from the environment are not primarily received and processed via this perception system, but rather from within the body itself.

Proprioception includes the perception of the position of our body in space, our movements, the positions of our joints and limbs, and the requirements needed to perform certain activities. Even when we are asleep, it plays a major role: otherwise, we would not be able to assess where we are in bed at any given moment and, in the worst case, would fall out because the distance to the edge would be too small.

Self-awareness can be divided into four areas:

1. **The sense of position**: we can sense where our limbs are even with our eyes closed or in the dark (i.e., without visual stimuli) and can, for example, easily move our right hand to our left knee.

2. **The sense of tension**: We can consciously influence our muscle tension. This enables us, for example, to maintain position during a handstand by dosing the body tension so that we neither overturn forward nor have to set down. A successfully executed cartwheel would also be due to the tension sense.

3. **The sense of force**: We can estimate how much muscle force must be applied for certain movements. For example, when we open a bag of our favorite candy, we have to apply just the right amount of force by pulling the wrapper apart so that a small hole can form, but it doesn't tear completely and everything falls out.

4. **The sense of movement**: We can determine the speed and direction of our movements even without visual contact with our limbs, for example when dancing.

It can therefore be stated that this system continuously provides detailed information and can work independently of visual impressions. The great importance of this is shown, for example, in the documentary "Our secret 6th sense", co-produced by Arte, which also deals with disorders of proprioception, among other things. According to their research, there are only 5 people in the world in whom this perceptual system fails. As a result, they do not know where their arms or legs are when they are not looking.

Every movement then requires a high degree of concentration and focus, yet injuries are inevitable because there is no sensation, which regulates the adjustment of tension and force application. Without visual contact, they are also unable to perform purposeful movements. Let's take climbing a spiral staircase as an example: someone with impaired proprioception would need to keep their foot in view to enable stepping onto the next step. After that, the gaze would have to move to the hand on the railing so that it can be carried along and provide stabilization. Climbing the steps in a fluid movement while holding on at the same time would not be possible.

This illustrates very vividly what we owe to our self-perception, even if most people have not been so aware of this until now.

The targeted training of self-awareness is accordingly important for competitive athletes, as it promotes movement coordination and helps them to learn and consolidate new reaction mechanisms. The better the information from inside the body is transmitted to our brain, the better the respective movement can be executed. The results of this training are clearly visible to everyone: for example, in professional figure skaters, every turn, every jump looks effortless and child's play, even though other people have trouble even staying on their feet on skates.

THE VESTIBULAR SYSTEM

But the fascinating functioning of our proprioception would be nothing without our vestibular system (lat. vestibulum = atrium, greek systema = compilation) - the sense of balance. What good is knowing where we are and how to move if we lack balance and can't walk straight, let alone stand?

This system is located in the inner ear and is located in the so-called petrous bone. Each ear therefore has a vestibular organ, which in turn has five core components:

• The **macular organs** sacculus and utriculus are responsible for processing linear movements of the head, i.e. forward/backward, up/down, left/right. This is done by registering changes in velocity in the respective direction, although these do not have to be triggered by head movements. We are known to register them as well, for example, when we are in a moving elevator or accelerating while driving a car.

• The **three arcuates** (anterior, posterior and horizontal), in turn, add to this information rotational movements that cover every possible angle to which we can move the head. As an example of external stimulation by a change in speed, we can list here, for example, a carousel in which we rotate in a circle.

This leads to the conclusion that our vestibular system reacts to accelerations of the head in a certain direction. This also enables protective reactions, since, for example, in the event of a fall, where our head moves rapidly downwards, the muscles are reflexively tensed shortly before impact. The body is thus cushioned and injuries are prevented as far as possible.

Furthermore, it is also responsible for stabilizing the image information that is transmitted through the eyes to the brain. For example, when we run forward, this is always associated with an up and down movement of the head - if our vestibular system were not functioning optimally, this would cause the images to blur before our eyes.

The three so-called vestibular reflexes are responsible for these different tasks:

1. **The vestibulo-spinal reflex**: This controls our posture in response to head movements and is the

cornerstone of our ability to stand or walk without difficulty. In addition, it also stabilizes our neck and cervical muscles as a support for our head and reacts with a countermovement when our body turns to help stabilize our gaze axis.

2. **The vestibulo-ocular reflex**: It ensures that our eyes move in the opposite direction to our head so that fixed objects remain in the field of vision. Look around once in your environment and then focus on a specific thing. Now turn your head in any direction and you may find that your eyes will not leave that thing, no matter where you turn your head and how fast (as long as it stays within reason, of course). However, if you notice dizziness, a blurred image, or even gait unsteadiness when you move quickly, this indicates a disorder of this reflex that should be treated.

3. **The vestibular nystagmus**: this reflex is similar to the vestibulo-ocular reflex just mentioned and regulates the slow eye movement opposite to the movement of the head in order to maintain our original field of vision.

However, it does not deal with the focus on a specific, fixed object, but with the general view through space. Just before the maximum deflection, there is a small corrective movement that allows us to turn our head further. Now look ahead, this is the field of view you want to focus on briefly. Slowly turn your head to one side without losing sight of the field of view. You will notice that this becomes more and more difficult with the increasing rotation and how your eyes will automatically jump a little bit further just before they stop, in order to expand the field of vision again.

Now, when it comes to training our balance, one probably first thinks of creating an uneven surface, a purposeful instability to which the body must then adapt. Wobble boards, mats or balls come into play. But before starting such exercises, one should first become aware of the cause of the lack of balance. This begins, like all other processes, in our brain. This controls our ability to postular control, that is, the ability to maintain our posture under the influence of gravity. This control is achieved by adjusting muscle tension to the appropriate requirements at any given time, thereby automatically balancing our body, whether we are in a static posture (i.e. standing) or in a dynamic movement.

In this way, a fluid equilibrium is established that constantly balances the forces acting on the body: The internal forces, i.e. our own movements, are oriented to the external forces, i.e. gravity and other circumstances, e.g. the nature of the ground. The center of gravity is shifted accordingly with each new movement so that we do not have to forfeit any of our freedom of movement.

Therefore, individual balance training should always start with optimizing our neuronal processes and functions before focusing primarily on external influences.

THE VISUAL SYSTEM

Last but not least is the visual system (lat. videre, visum = to see), which is mainly located in our eyes and enables us to visually perceive our environment in the first place. Vision involves up to 34 areas of our brain, which makes it so important for controlling our movements: it is assumed that between 60 and 80 percent of our movement designs depend on the information that our visual system takes in and processes.

The structure of the complete system is highly complex, as it includes all organic and nervous components involved in the reception and processing of optical impressions. We can roughly divide it into two components:

1. **The eye as an optical apparatus**. Its components include, for example, the lens, the vitreous body and the retina. Here, the lens focuses the light that passes through the cornea and the pupil and projects it onto the back of the eye. There, the retina can now generate a sharp image from it. The retina contains rod and cone cells that react to different light stimuli. Rods detect differences in brightness and enable us to see at dusk and at night as well as to see movement. Cones, on the other hand, are responsible for color perception and for enabling us to see our surroundings sharply.

2. **The neural part of** the visual system. In the retina there are ganglion cells, which in turn pass into the optic nerve. From here, the transmission of information via the visual pathway begins - the nerve first directs

the data towards the brain, where they are then processed further in the visual cortex and parts of the cerebral cortex. A part of the nerve cells of our retina ends in the pituitary gland, where the reflexes of our eyes are regulated, for example the pupil dilatation depending on the incidence of light. The other nerve strands cross each other, so this means that the information from the left eye is processed in the right hemisphere of the brain and vice versa.

Many different processes are responsible for the quality of this processed information, which in turn are largely dependent on the neurological nature of our eyes, nerves, and ultimately the other two movement-controlling entities: These include, for example, the functionality of our vestibular system (especially the vestibulo-ocular reflex), the coordination of our 12 eye muscles by the cerebellum, and the neuromechanical quality of our optic nerve.

But the great importance of our visual system can also bring equally great disadvantages, which is especially evident in competitive athletes: Our brain, as you have already learned, must make a danger assessment in every situation. This is done largely through visual stimuli, as these are the most direct and meaningful connection between our brain and our environment. To do this, it needs as much and as high quality information as possible. If this stimulus reception or transmission is even slightly disturbed, this can have far-reaching effects: The brain can now no longer make this prediction reliably, and performance is capped.

To counteract this problem, it is essential to check our eyes - however, it is not enough to go to the doctor regularly and have our vision checked. Targeted eye training is also necessary because, in addition to simply being able to assess our surroundings, it also helps us to do so as quickly as possible and thus be able to react optimally. A well-developed visual system is particularly important in team sports. For example, when running, soccer players have to keep a close eye on their surroundings and the other players at the same time in order to decide who to pass the ball to next or whether it makes more sense to try to score a goal themselves. They can't think for long, because some decisions have to be made in a fraction of a second in order to achieve the best possible result for the team.

Eye training should therefore achieve the following results in athletes:

• well controllable eye movements,

• an optimal dovetailing with proprioception: the athlete should be able to reliably assess his position in space as well as the depth relation to objects in his environment.

• visual clarity and

• good peripheral perception, i.e. the ability to recognize things that are at the edge of our field of vision.

The latter provides slightly distorted impressions and lower visual acuity, but movements are perceived much more efficiently. If something or someone suddenly appears at the edge of our field of vision, this new information is prioritized over the impressions that are directly in front of us and we direct our attention to it. It is believed that 98% of our visual information is blurred, that is, it occurs at the edge of our field of view. This has its origins in evolution, as our ancestors lived in constant danger. Since our sharp field of vision only covers a small part of our immediate surroundings, it was therefore particularly important to be able to notice things that were not happening directly in front of us. Without peripheral vision, many situations would have meant certain death, as an approaching enemy would not have been seen in time. In the meantime, the circumstances of life have changed completely, but this ability is still essential for our safety.

The implementation of eye training for spectacle wearers is also interesting. It is recommended to do it without glasses, because they always mean a visual restriction. The glasses thereby divide our field of vision into sharp and (significantly) blurred when we look beyond the edges. Since this disturbs us, we try to avoid it and rather turn our head in the desired direction to be able to see everything sharply. However, as a result, we use our eye muscles less, they become weaker and harder to coordinate. This can also affect our posture and the quality of our movements. Therefore, people who wear glasses should generally always resort to eye training in order to still benefit their eyes despite low vision and not make the situation even worse - regardless of whether they are athletes or not. You can also use contact lenses to make full use of your entire field of vision. However, if these aren't an option for you and you're too limited to train without visual aids, then put on your glasses. After all, limited training is better than no training.

In summary, each of the three instances does very impressive work and lays the foundation for the daily experience and exploration of our environment. Nevertheless, they are always dependent on the cooperation of the others: You can think of each instance as a cogwheel in this regard. Although they are mature and functional on their own, they are only able to rotate properly and unfold their full effect when they are interlocked and interconnected.

The focus of neuroathletics training should therefore not only be on a specific problem or system, which may require special attention. Rather, all instances should be considered and trained so that they can further promote each other.

Do not forget to warm up

Now that you have learned a lot about the structure and functioning of our nervous system, it is time to put this into practice.

Even if "only" our brain is being trained and we do not need to warm up with dynamic stretching exercises, loose running in or warm-up sets with lighter weights, it is recommended to prepare our brain for the upcoming training as well. Our brain as well as our mind should be receptive and able to work in a concentrated manner. However, if you regularly have a head full and your thoughts are racing from problem to problem, this should be the focus first and a solution should be found. Whether the electricity bill has already been paid, the car needs to be inspected again, or when you will be able to see your friends again despite your busy schedule are important aspects of your life that you cannot simply push into the background, but care should be taken to ensure that these questions do not occupy you incessantly and thus prevent you from relaxing once in a while. Mental relaxation in particular is so important for your training, as you want to focus on the correct execution of the exercises in order to really achieve the desired results.

In order to help you with this targeted, temporary letting go of your problems, we are now going to look at a few tips that are primarily aimed at the following two aspects: Your mental health and the physiological health of your brain as an organ.

However, mental health is not only the absence of a mental disorder, but also the state of general well-being. In addition to sports, there are other ways to promote it. Some examples:

1. **Write down your thoughts**. This can be done in a diary, a blog, or even using the note function on your phone. On the one hand, you don't run the risk of forgetting important or promising thoughts in the hustle

and bustle of everyday life, and on the other hand, you also support the brain in this way, because by writing it down you give it a sign that this particular thing is important. This specifically prevents it from being inadvertently classified by the brain as unimportant and pushed into the background, if not forgotten. From now on, you can organize your everyday life more stress-free and have everything important on call when it is needed.

2. **Find a hobby to freely express your creativity**. We spend most of our day with rationality and logic, we usually have rigid ways of working and strict guidelines to which we have to adhere. This also limits our way of thinking, we develop a kind of tunnel vision over time. Give yourself time off from this regularly and find something that fulfills you: Paint a picture, sing and dance, write a short story. You don't have to be perfect or necessarily please others, nor do you have to have a goal. The main thing is that you have fun.

3. **Meditate**. Whether through a yoga class or a seated meditation in silence, you will notice the positive effects after a short time. This way, you specifically train your mind to simultaneously allow complete

silence to enter your thoughts and, on the other hand, to direct your full attention to a specific thing, such as your breathing or a sound from the environment.

You can do the meditation freely according to your ideas or follow a guided one, where you are instructed step by step. The only important thing is that you do it without time pressure and that you are ready to open your mind.

4. **Unplug**. We're used to being under constant pressure: The phone is often at our fingertips, and for some, an uneasy feeling creeps in when we're not constantly reachable. Social media accompanies us at every turn, as we want to be connected and keep up with the lives of our friends or even the stars we can't reach. As a result, however, we increasingly compare ourselves with others, and this illusory world promotes pressure to perform and envy. Consciously take the time to focus on the essentials again.

Once you've fulfilled your purpose for the day, turn off your phone, step outside and enjoy the beautiful sights you miss when your eyes are glued to your screen. Take a walk with your loved ones and enjoy the here and now.

5. **Schedule time for yourself in your schedule**. Many people tend to always think of other people's needs first and come up short themselves. Whether it's at work or in family life, there's always something to do. But don't forget yourself in this hustle and bustle, because you don't live only for others. Everyone can sacrifice at least 5 minutes a day to take care of themselves.

So take this time and then do what you want. Read a book, take care of your body and take a long bath, watch an episode of your favorite show or just lie on the couch if you feel like it. This time is completely yours, so don't let it interfere or influence you.
So try a little and find out what helps you feel good.

Now, in order to do something good for the brain not only on a psychological but also on a physical level, you should also pay attention to the following:

• Sufficient and quality sleep.
We sleep for about one third of our lives, which is why we should by no means underestimate its importance. Sleep primarily serves to regenerate and repair our brain. However, this can only take place during this time, as our nervous system would be overwhelmed by this while awake - after all, you can't maintain a train at full speed at the same time. So in order for your brain

to be able to optimally process all the information from the previous day and for you to start the next day fully refreshed, you should aim to sleep between 7 and 8 hours every night.

To get the most out of your sleep, there are a few key things you should consider:

1. You should (if possible) have a <u>regular sleep rhythm</u>, i.e. always go to bed at about the same time and get up the next morning. This ensures that your body automatically gets tired at the same time out of habit, in preparation for the sleep to come. You thus avoid going to bed and still lying awake for a long time.

2. Create your <u>own individual sleep ritual</u>. This ensures peace and relaxation in the time before you actually go to bed and helps you find your way to sleep even more easily. You can take your preferences into account: Popular sleep rituals include listening to music or reading. However, you should focus on not putting your brain through too much more. Rather, use light and relaxing sounds or reading. If you are used to falling asleep with a running TV in the background, it would be better to play an audio book or white noise, rain sounds, etc. instead. The flickering light of the TV

as well as the sometimes strongly fluctuating volume could disturb the course of the sleep phases.

3. <u>Writing down your experiences of the day</u> can also help you to briefly review the impressions and then conclude with them.

4. <u>Breathing exercises and relaxation exercises</u> are also very beneficial for the process of falling asleep and additionally help to train the sensitivity for tensions in your own body - sometimes you realize that you have been holding certain muscle groups tense for a long time without realizing it (e.g. tense jaw, contracted eyebrows).

5. Also, make sure <u>not to exercise 2 to 3 hours before bedtime,</u> otherwise your circulation and metabolism will still be too stimulated to wind down. The same time mark also applies to <u>eating larger meals</u>, otherwise the still-working digestion can disturb our sleep.

6. If you like, you can also try <u>autosuggestion.</u> This involves mentally telling yourself certain things, such as *"I am tired,"* *"My body is completely relaxed,"* and *"I am now letting go of all tension.* Sounds a bit strange, but it

works as long as you are really convinced of this statement and do not doubt it or say it only as a means to an end. If you do this with the complete belief that what you are saying really applies to you, then you are training your subconscious mind. This part of our psyche cannot otherwise be directly influenced or addressed by us, but it itself has a great influence on our lives.

It ensures that many processes run automatically so as not to overtax our brain (otherwise we would have to think specifically about every single blink and every breath, for example) and learns in the process through regular repetition. So if you tell yourself often enough to be relaxed, over time your subconscious will ensure that you will no longer be prone to such unrecognized, tense postures and will automatically relax more. You will actually be able to fall asleep more easily.

• **Brain Food**:

Provide your brain with enough important nutrients and make sure you eat a healthy, balanced diet. Here, too, there are some tips and certain foods that are particularly effective, as well as some habits to avoid.

This is especially important because many people now do jobs that do not require strenuous physical activity, but rather mental activity. For many hours a day, you have to solve problems, remember important data and be able to recall it at any time. Tiredness, headaches and impaired receptivity are often the result. To avoid this in the future as best as possible, you should actively support your brain with a good supply of nutrients.

If you notice that your brain functions drop for a short time, this is often due to a lack of trace elements such as potassium, selenium and zinc. You can replenish this store with pears, nuts, garlic or spinach, for example.

But nuts are not only rich in trace elements, but also contain important E and B vitamins and unsaturated (healthy) fatty acids. These strengthen our memory and nerve function, and also make us learn better. However, make sure to eat nuts only in moderation, as they are very high in calories. As a small snack between meals, they are very suitable, especially as a substitute for chips or gummy bears. Broccoli, fish, strawberries or avocados also improve your brain health.

We should also pay equal attention to the type of food we eat and how we eat it:

1. <u>Eat regularly</u>. Few and lavish meals can make us sluggish, the body has to spend a lot of energy on digestion, and we need time before we feel fit and able to perform again. In addition, the blood sugar level drops if there is too much time between meals. However, since this should remain as constant as possible for optimal brain performance, we should also supply our body with nutrients in between meals. It's up to you whether you split your meals according to your calorie requirements and eat five meals instead of three, for example, or whether you pack yourself healthy snacks (primarily fruit or vegetables).

Bananas are an excellent snack because, in addition to important nutrients such as magnesium, they contain complex carbohydrates that cause our blood sugar levels to rise and fall only slowly. With simple carbohydrates, such as highly sugary sweets, blood sugar shoots up, giving us a short-term energy boost. However, this drops again just as quickly afterwards, resulting in fatigue and a lack of concentration.

2. Also, make sure to consume <u>as few processed foods</u> or meals <u>as possible.</u> A frozen pizza is delicious and quick to prepare. Especially when you come home from work after a long day, it sounds like a tempting alternative to cooking. However, appearances are deceiving - for example, the "ham" that is advertised large on the package is often only 50 to 90 percent real meat. The rest is filler and water. In addition, highly processed foods are usually loaded with lots of sugar, fat, salt and preservatives. Coloring agents and stabilizers are also often found on the ingredients list - after all, the ready-made food is supposed to look nicely presented and appetizing. However, this not only adds unnecessary substances to your body, but also many more calories than you would have consumed with a meal prepared by yourself.

3. But if you do need to go fast, you can use <u>meal</u> prepping as an alternative to cooking - that is, pre-cooking various dishes for several days so that you always have a complete meal available and only have to heat it up when hunger strikes.

But again, this is very time consuming. If it doesn't fit into your schedule, next time you prepare your favorite dish, why not cook a little more on purpose and freeze it to enjoy later?

4. So in general, try to <u>cook</u> more. This not only saves money, but is also fun and there are countless dishes for every level of requirement and diet. In an ideal meal, the three macronutrients protein, carbohydrates and fats should be balanced on our plate. Approximately one-third should be filled with a protein source such as fish or chicken; as a reference size, you can use the size and thickness of your own palm. The remaining two-thirds should be filled with carbohydrates that have a low glycemic index, such as quinoa, whole grain pasta or bread, vegetables and lettuce. The fats can be taken either as 1 tsp of oil (olive oil, linseed oil or similar) spread over the meal or by adding avocado or nuts.

5. Also, eat <u>breakfast,</u> even if this is sometimes difficult to reconcile with individual daily rhythms. Some people are simply not hungry early in the morning. In this case, you should not force yourself to eat an extensive breakfast of toast, scrambled eggs and juice.

But if you're used to a morning cup of coffee to start your day, why not eat a light snack with it, such as a homemade fruit salad or even some natural yogurt or skyr. This will give your brain and the rest of your body enough energy and performance to get going and make good use of the morning.

In addition, you should always drink enough, because even a small fluid deficit can mean fatigue and difficulty concentrating. The optimal amount per day is 2 to 2.5 liters, it should never be less than 1.5 liters. If you have problems reaching this amount, a regular reminder on your cell phone or even a motivational bottle can help. These usually show the respective number of milliliters at regular intervals, as well as a time at which you should have already consumed this amount of fluid. However, as far as possible, avoid drinks with a high sugar content, such as soft drinks, juices or excessive consumption of alcohol. Priority should be given to water (with or without sparkling water), highly diluted juices or unsweetened tea.

Try to integrate some of these tips into your life in the best possible way. Your brain will now be more receptive and efficient, which will provide the optimal basis for the upcoming training.

Get Started

You are now well informed and ready to start neuroathletics training.

However, before you can start with the actual exercises, it is important to get a rough overview of the state of your nervous system. The training can only develop its full effect if you know where your deficits are and where you need to start in order to remedy them.

You achieve this through the strategy of "testing and retesting". You first perform a basic exercise that you observe with regard to a specific aspect: This can be, for example, the conversion of your strength or the number of repetitions during strength training, but also your mobility, balance or focus.

For example, perform a standing balance, so stand up straight and lean forward as far as you can while extending both arms and one leg. Try to balance and keep the body as level as possible. Now perform any exercise from neuroathletics training. For example, it would be a good idea to look for a fixed point at eye level, then fixate on it at all times while bobbing up and down. This primarily appeals to our vestibular system, which now takes over the task of stabilizing our gaze during this rocking movement. After about 60 seconds, you now perform a standing balance again and evaluate the difference from before:

Do you find the exercise easier and feel more stable, is it neutral and no change can be noticed, or do you find it more difficult? In the latter case, your nervous system is now signaling to you that it has difficulty assessing the situation and is therefore switching to safety mode to protect you from injury. This is exactly this unconscious throttling of your performance, which we have covered before and which needs to be recognized. You have now identified a weak point and know what you need to train especially in the coming weeks.

The most important thing is that after performing the neuroathletic exercise, you do not wait long before performing the test exercise. Our nervous system reacts immediately to this new information and you will see the results immediately, unlike a conventional physical exercise. Waiting time would thus only distort the results. But don't get too fired up by the quick results, regular training is still necessary to achieve long-term improvement. Recommended is 20 to 30 minutes of intensive neuroathletic training daily. However, if your nervous system is initially overwhelmed by this many additional influences and you feel unwell, it is better to split the time into 4 to 6 smaller units of 5 minutes each, which you complete over the course of the day.

You should also follow these principles:

• Our movement-controlling systems are so closely interconnected that you automatically train all of them with one exercise, even if the focus is on the sense of balance, for example. Nevertheless, you are subject to a hierarchy through your respective share in our information collection and formation:

The visual system is at the top, followed by the vestibular system and finally the proprioception. It therefore makes sense to also train from top to bottom so that the other two are warmed up via the visual system and optimally prepared for the following stress.

However, this is not a must. It can also happen that your eyes are quickly overloaded at the beginning of your new routine and your body reacts strongly to the visual training, for example in the form of dizziness or blurred vision. So if you get uncomfortable, follow the hierarchy from bottom to top to warm up your eyes. So go slow and follow your body's signals. The NAT should not cause discomfort or pain at any time.

• If you experience positive feedback from your brain one day during an exercise, but suddenly experience negative feedback the next day, don't be upset. You are not doing anything wrong with your training. These differences are due to the fact that, just like the rest of our bodies, the circumstances for our brains vary each day. One day you're in top shape and could be pulling out trees, the next day you may have had trouble slee-ping or you may have been feeding your body too few nutrients, resulting in poorer performance.

These fluctuations are normal. On such days, simply concentrate on other exercises that show you other weak points again - neuroathletics training should be flexible and not follow a rigid sequence that always consists of the same tasks. After all, the brain always wants to be challenged anew and not just get used to the influences.

It is worthwhile to perform testing and retesting with each neuroathletic exercise that you want to include in your training. To supplement this, it is best to create an overview on which you note the respective exercise, the result and the date. Check and compare your notes at regular intervals, such as every 2 weeks. For better clarification, you can also film yourself performing the exercises and compare your posture - you will not only feel a big difference from your self-awareness of your body behavior, but you will also be able to see it clearly from the outside. Alternatively, you can look for a training partner who will pay close attention to you. This doesn't necessarily require a trained trainer's eye, even lay people can often spot the differences when they observe you.

Most of the neuroathletics training exercises can be completed without equipment, but the following tools are needed:

- A ruler, pencil, or your fingers: For most tasks, you need at least one fixed point that you should always focus on during execution (which again illustrates the enormous part our eyes play in controlling movement). The most common is any letter, because letters are much faster and easier to recognize when our vision becomes blurry, which is why opticians often use them in eye tests. You can write this letter on a ruler, a pen or on a fingernail. Alternatively, you can print it on a piece of paper and attach it to a wall, but the other options are usually more effective. To adjust the difficulty, simply increase (easier) or decrease (harder) the letter.

- Should you want to integrate more challenging methods into your training plan after some time, then exercise balls or wobble boards can help. This intentional creation of an unstable surface provides your brain with completely new impressions and further builds on your previous progress. However, before doing so, you should make sure that your individual instances are well trained and that the nervous system feels safe enough to engage in these new situations with full power.

- Resistance bands. These additionally help your brain to control the movements.

Now pick specific exercises that you are comfortable with and start testing and retesting.

Here is an exemplary overview of how you can easily test the individual motion-controlling systems:

• **Visual System**: Since most of our visual input is through our peripherals, it makes the most sense to use them for testing. Find a training partner to help you with this.

Now perform a specific task that you are confident in. This could be juggling or jumping rope, for example. First perform the exercise normally for a while until you have become well acquainted with the movement sequence. Now rate on a scale of 1 to 10 how easy it was for you to perform the exercise.

Start the exercise again, because now your partner comes into play, positioning himself to the side of you and alternately pointing up a different number of fingers. Continue to concentrate completely on the task, your gaze does not deviate to your partner's hand. Along the way, say aloud the numbers that are being shown to you. Pause briefly after 30 to 60 seconds, your partner can now stand again so that he has a good view of you. Now perform the basic exercise one last time and re-evaluate the ease of execution. Your partner may also be able to see a change and confirm your view. Make a note of the result.

• **Vestibular system**: One of the main tasks of our vestibular system is gaze stabilization, visual acuity should be ensured with every conceivable head movement. Again, look for your partner, because they can notice the possible fluttering of your eyes much faster and more clearly than you can.

In the following exercise, we test the horizontal arc by turning the head to the right or left: You first need your letter, i.e. pen/ruler/finger. Now stretch one arm forward and hold the letter at about the level of your eyes. Focus on it while turning your head so that it is just possible for both eyes to see the letter. Now close your eyes and slowly (you should need about 5 seconds for the movement) bring your head back to the center. Repeat this process five to ten times with each side. If the letter becomes blurred, this indicates deficits in your vestibular system.

- **Proprioceptive system**: There are numerous ways to test your self-perception. Take your depth perception, for example: The idea here is to observe whether you can perform a certain movement comparably with your eyes open and with them closed, or whether your muscle posture deviates greatly when the visual input is removed. Film the movement or have someone observe you. Now stretch your right arm to the right away from your body, bring it up so that it is vertical next to your head, and then forward until it is at a right angle to the rest of your body. Finally, from there you can bring it back to the starting position to the right, creating a fluid movement that is best repeated a few times with each arm. With your eyes closed, this should usually look very similar.

You could also test depth perception, for example, by standing in front of a wall at some distance, now dropping forward and intercepting yourself. Even with your eyes closed, your body should be able to intuitively recognize how much space remains to the wall and when you need to extend your hands to prevent a collision.

Now you know the basis to explore your nervous system with all its weak points and also strengths. The following list contains various neuroathletic training exercises that will then help you work through your deficits and strengthen each movement-controlling system.

- **Train your visual system**:
    - o <u>Eye tracking</u>: Use your letter to help you. Focus on it, then move your tool in an H-shape, i.e. linearly. From the starting point, it first goes up, then down, then back to the center. After that, move it to the left or right and repeat the movement to get the letter H. Do this a few times and intensify the exercise by increasing the speed. However, the rule is that you must still be able to see the letter sharply at all times. If you feel comfortable with this exercise, add circular movements: trace a spiral. Either start at a short distance from your face, then paint the spiral larger and larger and move away, or vice versa.

o <u>Accommodation</u>: In addition to your letter, find another object that is about 5 to 20 meters away from you. Now alternately focus on the letter (sometimes hold it so close to your eyes that you have to squint) and the object in the background. A similar task is also recommended for people who spend most of their working day in front of a screen: the 20:20 exercise, in which you look at something 20 meters away every 20 minutes. A longer look out of the window is usually enough to relax your eyes.

o <u>Fixation</u>: To do this, print or draw a square on a sheet of paper. It is easiest if each corner of the square is connected to every other corner, i.e. the diagonal lines are also visible. You can also highlight the center of the square. First, fix the center, then let your gaze wander from there to each corner and follow each line with your gaze. In this way, you additionally train the eye muscle, since we are often no longer used to moving our eyes exclusively. For example, if we want to look down at our phone, we tilt our head rather than just lowering our gaze and minimize the actual work of our eyes. This is especially important for people who wear glasses, to break out of this "cage" that the glasses represent for our field of vision every now and then.

o <u>Eye jumps</u>: You now need two tools with letters. The letter must be the same and both should also be the same size. Now hold one aid in each hand and stretch out your arms. These should then be at a 45° angle to each other, with the letters at eye level. Your gaze initially leads straight ahead, i.e. between the fixed points. Now look to the left, focus on the letter and then jump over to the other one. The head always remains straight and does not move. Repeat this several times and feel free to experiment with the speed - but here, too, the motto is that the letter must first be in focus before you continue.

o Your visual system can also be trained by <u>activat-ing the VOR</u>, or vestibulo-ocular reflex. You will learn exactly how this works in the next point.

- **Exercises for the** vestibular **system:**
  o <u>Infinity Walk</u>: To do this, you walk around the infinity sign or an 8. You can delimit this by any two objects, for example two balls, which you then circle alternately. Now look for a fixed point at eye level, which can be either directly in your line of sight or to the side of you, so that you have to walk sideways. Now first try to fix this point while walking the 8 without having to look at your gait or making mistakes. To increase, you can switch from walking to jogging or running, dribbling a ball or even running backwards. However, since this exercise is generally not easy, you should start slowly.

  o <u>Stimulate the macular organs</u>: To do this, place a letter at eye level, your distance to it should be one arm's length. Fix it in place and bob up and down as you do so. Start with a neutral head posture, the gaze is directed straight ahead. Now, to reach the sacculus and utriculus completely, you need to cause a linear acceleration of the head. To do this, now turn your head to the left and right, keeping your eyes on the letter as usual. Then turn it forward again and bring the chin slightly to the chest. Rocking with the head hyperextended, i.e. tilted upward, should be done at the end, as this hyperextension puts additional stress on the nervous system. Only build this into your workout if the previous movements could be performed safely and without problems.

If you want to work your vestibular system even harder, eliminate the visual stimuli by repeating the exercises with your eyes closed.

o <u>Don't forget the arches</u>: now stretch out your arms at a 45° angle, your thumbs pointing up. These will serve as your fixed points again in a moment. Pull your chin slightly toward your chest, fix one thumb, and then move your head to the other every second (as long as it is sharply detected in one second). The head movement here must be done quickly, as the vestibular system responds to the change in speed. Do this for 15 to 20 times per side. The rotation of the head here activates the arcuate pathways. To cover all 3 of these, you can then hold one arm higher than the other to exercise the diagonals as well. Repeat this with each side as well.

o Stand upright, your fixed point should be at eye level. Fix this and now tilt your head alternately from front to back without releasing your gaze. If the letter cannot be held sharply, try a larger one. Again, problems can occur due to the hyperextension of the head, which is why you should only perform the exercise at rest and not before another, physical workout. If you feel sick or uncomfortable, then only continue slowly and carefully or leave the exercise out for the time being.

o You can also take your tool at hand and fix it from an arm's length away, walking forward or backward.

• Promote proprioception:

This is probably the system that is easiest to train, because it is stimulated by every single movement. A few examples would be:

o <u>Sensory warm-up</u>: The aim here is to trigger the mechanoreceptors on our skin. You can achieve this, for example, by rolling the entire body over a fascia roller. This rolling movement over the individual muscles, bones and joints helps the brain to register their position in relation to each other in a more targeted manner, which is also a very effective aid for an upcoming workout: First perform a testing and retesting with any stretching exercise. The intermediate unrolling will increase your nervous system's sense of safety, which in turn will increase pain and stretch tolerance. Consequently, you will be able to hold the stretch longer and deeper than before.

o <u>Walking barefoot in the sand</u>: thereby train your body to adapt to this new and still relatively unknown surface. It must now develop a new sense of stability and balance so that you can walk safely.

o <u>Walking with eyes closed</u>: Due to the lack of visual input, you now have to rely on your depth perception. Try walking along a straight line. Take a training partner to help you with this, who can judge the results.

o <u>Stability training</u>: Here, resort to one-arm or one-leg exercises. This can be a Plank, where you extend one arm out to the side after turning in stability, forcing you to use the other arm to hold yourself stable and adjust your body's center of gravity. Other examples would be Pistol Squats, standing balances, or single-leg Glute Bridges.

o <u>Use resistance</u>: If you have resistance bands, you can also use them to improve your self-awareness. For example, fix the band under one foot and then stretch it over the shoulder of the same side. Now perform a few squats slowly and with concentration. The stretching of the band and the additional pull will result in higher control requirements for your movement control than if you were to perform the exercise freely. The band will guide you as the cerebellum controls the movement at all times to prevent injury. Go slow, letting your nervous system register that there is no danger. This allows it to become accustomed to doing the exercise correctly, and you are less likely to risk instability or poor posture later if you omit the band.

To improve proprioception, it is also recommended to train your hands specifically:

1. Perform what is called a <u>Flexion Wave</u>:

Angle one arm in front of your body, your forearm should be perpendicular and parallel to your torso, and your thumb should be facing you so that you can see your hand from the side. Keep it stiff at first and start curling your fingers slowly, limb by limb. Now, when your fingertips touch your palm (this should happen at about the base of your fingers), try to maintain contact with it. Don't curl your fingers any further, you don't want to make a fist, but stroke the tips away down along the palm. Once you have reached the lowest point, bring your fingers forward away from your hand, bend them upward in a sweeping motion, and return them to the starting position. Performed quickly, the movement resembles a wave, hence the appropriate name. This may be a bit difficult and uncomfortable the first few times, but you'll get used to it and in turn get a better feel for your fingers.

2. <u>Extension Wave:</u> This works like the Flexion Wave, but in reverse. Start with the same arm position, your fingertips touching your palm at its lower edge. Now let them slide upwards and try to maintain contact with the palm for as long as possible.

3. The previous two exercises can also be done with the <u>thumb.</u> Stretch it away from the hand at a 90-degree angle, then curve it and slowly guide it along the palm before bringing it forward away from it again. The thumb should leave the palm at about the level of the pinky finger. For the Extension Wave, simply perform this movement backwards again.

4. <u>Mobilize your fingers</u>: To do this, stretch your hand out horizontally in front and spread your fingers. You can start with any finger, but the index finger is recommended. Now touch it on the upper and lower side with the thumb and index finger of your other hand

and find the joint that connects finger and hand.

This is not located directly on the knuckle, but a little lower in the direction of the palm. Move the finger to be trained up and down, you will clearly notice where exactly it is located. Now fix the joint with your thumb and index finger, because you want to make sure that the following movements originate from it and additionally mobilize it. To begin with, move the fixed finger linearly, either from left to right or from top to bottom. If this doesn't cause you any problems, then draw small circles. Repeat these exercises several times as well as in all directions, working your way from finger to finger.

These exercises help your brain learn how to better control the individual fingers in isolation from each other. Future movements that focus on our hands become more predictable (for example, doing a handstand or passing a ball). In everyday life, most of the focus is usually only on the thumb and index finger, so training the other fingers can give you an additional performance boost.

As mentioned, this list is not exhaustive, but it contains the most important tasks you need to start your training.

10-week plan with which you can optimally incorporate neuroathletics training into your everyday life

Putting together the best routine for you from these numerous exercises and already thinking of everything important at the beginning is not easy and requires a precise overview. The following 10-week plan should serve you as a basic framework for getting started and help you to be able to concentrate completely on the exercises.

Since each person has a different neurological profile and, accordingly, different requirements, you still need to adjust the plan a little to get the best result for you. It is therefore kept as general as possible and considers all movement-controlling instances equally. However, customization should not be a problem due to the testing and retesting explained earlier. Just add the exercises to the plan that will benefit you the most.

At the end of the 10 weeks, you will feel much more confident in using the neuroathletic training and can now decide if you feel ready for the more challenging exercises with the integrated balance training or continue training without the equipment.

• **Week 1 - Preparation**

In the first week, the focus is not yet on the training itself, but on optimal preparation. It's best to create a checklist so that you don't lose track of everything. You will need:

1. Your <u>personal tool</u> with the letter that will serve as your visual fixed point during a large part of the exercises. If you prefer to use a ruler or pen instead of writing on your fingernails, prepare several tools and letters of different sizes in advance so that you can adjust the difficulty if necessary.

2. A <u>(cell phone) camera or your training partner</u> <u>who is available</u> to you for a few minutes each day.

3. <u>Sturdy shoes</u>. Normal sports shoes are perfectly adequate. You want to make sure you have as secure a footing as possible, especially at the beginning of training, so that you can get an unbiased impression of your abilities during testing.

4. <u>Loose clothing</u>. Since you will sometimes want to perform movements with a larger radius, your clothes should not constrict you in the process.

5. Your personal <u>training diary</u>. Create an overview of your progress and document your training in detail. Where and how you do it doesn't matter, the main thing is that you have it quickly at hand and it is well structured.

6. <u>Reflect</u> on your previous habits. Are you perhaps eating too unbalanced, are you permanently stressed and neglecting yourself? Then pick out a few delicious, healthy recipes, make a note of the ingredients on your shopping list and try, step by step, to promote your mental health.

7. <u>Create workout times</u>. Your schedule is bursting at the seams and you can't find a coherent half hour in which to complete your exercises? Then split up the units, but keep track of them. It would be a good idea to make it your goal to exercise for 5 minutes every 1.5 h until you have reached the total time. If need be, have your phone remind you if this gets lost in the stress of everyday life. Some tasks can

also be done perfectly from your desk (like the 20:20 exercise mentioned earlier) and additionally help you to switch off briefly and relieve your eyes.

- ***Week 2 - Start***

Optimally, you now have everything together and feel fit, so you can finally get started.

Slowly familiarize yourself with the execution of neuroathletic training and start testing yourself. However, don't overexert yourself and especially don't let yourself get stressed. You are just beginning to deal with your nervous system in a concrete way, so it is clear that you will not be able to recognize and classify every single connection immediately. You will develop a feeling for this over time; after all, no master has fallen from the sky yet.

You can aim for at least 3 to 5 minutes for one exercise, which is why you should not do more than 10 tests a day so as not to overtax your brain.

Starting with the visual system, that is, following the original hierarchy, your training sequence might then look like this:

- **Visual system:**
  - <u>Two tests of the periphery</u>: Together with your training partner, perform the exercise

described earlier, in which the partner shows you a changing number of his fingers while performing another task. After that, you can perform a so-called "bunny drill". In this, the partner positions himself behind you, shows bunny ears with his hands, and then lets them hop next to your head from back to front in your field of view. This involves dividing the field of view into four quadrants (top left and right, bottom left and right), which are worked through one at a time. As soon as you see the bunny, say "Hepp" loudly so that your partner knows. If this test reveals significant deficits in any of the quadrants, see a doctor. This could be due to a more serious illness that cannot be remedied with mere neuro athletic training.

- <u>A test of the sharp field of vision</u>: Take your letter in hand, hold it at eye level and fix it. Now alternately bring it closer to your eyes so that you have to squint and then move it further away again. This can also be repeated if you cover one eye at a time and thus assess each side separately.

- o **Vestibular System**:
  - ▪ Work here using the <u>bobbing motions</u>: Focus on the letter as you bob up and down. You can address the various components of your vestibular organ (i.e., the macular organs and the arcuate ducts) while doing this by using various head movements and rotations. So tilt your head to the side, pull your chin toward your chest, or turn your head slightly away. Feel free to vary a bit, but use both sides of your head equally. Don't forget: The ears each have an equal weight organ that needs to be stimulated accordingly.

- o **Proprioception**:
  - ▪ Perform <u>any three movement tests</u> with alternating open and closed eyes and have your partner observe you. Since our proprioception is stimulated by each individual movement, you have free choice when testing.

At the end of week 2, you should have a rough overview of where your deficits lie. Make a note of them and keep them in mind when selecting exercises in the future, as well as their weighting during training. You don't have to keep the 3/3/3 split, it's just important that you don't neglect any system.

• *Week 3 - Start of training*

Now it's time to start the actual training. Conduct a short test each day to determine individual requirements. However, don't spend too much time on this, as you now want to center on promoting the systems con and you don't want to drag out the training unnecessarily - after all, you don't want to overload your brain.

Again, work through the exercises according to the hierarchy from top to bottom or vice versa.

Before you start training, record 5 exercises per system. Then pick 3 exercises to do each day. You don't have to vary every day, but it is advisable to add a new stimulus every few days, which the brain then has to get used to - so it stays alert.

• *Week 4, 5 and 6 - training phase:*

After you have familiarized yourself with neuroathletics training in the 3rd week, the phase in which you can train without restrictions now begins. Continue your previous training plan, diligently complete your training diary and get to know your body better.

Choose 2 new exercises per week from the overview of the many different exercises that you integrate into your training from time to time. Don't let it become monotonous and challenge yourself consciously, for this you need new stimuli.

If you are not already doing so, then also incorporate coordination, stability or stretching exercises into your sports program at the same time. Light strength training will also have a positive effect on your development: If our brains are now learning to give the green light for full performance on a more regular basis, then it only makes sense to supplement this with an increase in our overall strength.

If you already play another sport, try to maintain the level over this time. It is still too early to make big leaps. First, consolidate your knowledge of neuroathletics and give your nervous system time to adapt and correct the deficits step by step - the results will be all the better for it in a few weeks.

• *Week 7 and 8 - Interim report*

You have now successfully trained your nervous system for the last 1.5 months and hopefully already noticed one or two small successes. Now take your diary and consciously take the time to leaf back to the beginning.

What differences do you notice? How far have you come so far? Feel free to write that down, too, because no matter how small the progress may be, it will motivate you to keep going.

For your sport (if any), you can now start pushing further to your limits. Take more weight, dare to try new movement patterns or use a different running route that includes more uneven ground or even inclines and declines. Closely observe your body's response.

Why don't you go hiking in the forest and explore nature from time to time as a supplement to your training and mental health efforts? The numerous new impressions and demands, in addition to the beautiful view, will challenge all movement-controlling systems, giving you a double success right away.
Diligently continue to complete your exercises and look to the future with motivation.

• *Week 9 - Almost* advanced

Now that you're already accustomed to the training routine, it's time to also incorporate some small stimuli into your normal daily life to help you develop.
Proprioceptive training is ideally suited for this purpose:

Stand on one leg more often, or challenge yourself to balance on a rolled up towel for the duration of your tooth brushing. A flexion wave is also quick to do. Exercise your hands regularly now, too; learn a handstand. Encourage your grip strength.

You might also get excited about new, strenuous tasks: try balancing on a slackline between two trees without falling.

Also, feel free to consider which exercises can still support your nervous system without looking at the overview. By now you have developed a sense of what your nervous system needs, how the individual tasks work and what they are aimed at. So feel free to develop your own exercise, because as long as it brings you closer to your goal, there are no limits to your creativity.

- ***Week 10 - From beginner to expert***

You have now reached the end of this plan and have laid the foundation for future athletic success as well as fully comprehensive training.

Now take your diary again and be proud of what you have already achieved. Reflect on whether you still have previous deficits and ask yourself what your focus is now. If you want to continue to eradicate your weak points, focus on work-up exercises as before.

These are the ones where you noticed during testing and retesting that you are having difficulty performing and you are being negatively affected. If you have already trained your nervous system so well that it is at a good level all around, and you additionally want to achieve new success in your respective favorite sport, shift your neuroathletics training to the time immediately before the sporting activity. In addition, you should resort to high-performance exercises here: These have been shown to greatly improve movement control when tested. They will help you build on previous progress and take your performance to a new level.

The last 10 weeks should have changed the way you feel completely: You feel more energetic, more confident in your movements and more utilized. You are hopefully feeling better both mentally and physically and have taken a liking to this healthier lifestyle.

Don't let up and train in the future as meticulously as before to continue living in optimal harmony with your nervous system. Challenge yourself regularly and test your new limits - you have long since left the old ones behind.

Now enjoy your new life and look forward to all that may come.